Copyright © 2019 k

All rights reserved. No part of this publication may be reproduced, distributed, or transmitted in any form or by any means, including photocopying, recording, or other electronic or mechanical methods, without the prior written permission of the publisher, except in the case of brief quotations embodied in critical reviews and certain other noncommercial uses permitted by copyright law.

# Contents

- INTRODUCTION .................................................................. 3
- PREGNANCY ....................................................................... 5
  - The Three Stages of Pregnancy (1st, 2nd, and 3rd Trimester) 7
    - First Trimester .................................................................. 7
    - Second Trimester ........................................................... 10
    - Third Trimester ............................................................... 13
  - Symptoms of Pregnancy ................................................... 17
    - Spotting and Cramping .................................................. 18
    - Breast Changes ............................................................... 19
    - Fatigue ............................................................................ 20
    - Nausea (Morning Sickness) ........................................... 20
    - Missed Period ................................................................. 21
  - Causes of pregnancy ......................................................... 22
  - Diagnosis ............................................................................ 25
- OKRA ................................................................................... 30
  - The Benefits Of Okra During Pregnancy ......................... 30
    - Nutritional Value Of Okra .............................................. 33
- OKRA FOR PREGNANT WOMAN ......................................... 35
  - Ways to Include Okra in Pregnancy Diet ........................ 36
  - Dosage ................................................................................ 36
  - Side Effects ........................................................................ 38

# INTRODUCTION

Okra (Abelmoschus esculentus L.) is an important vegetable grown for its green tender fruits which are used as a vegetable in a variety of ways. It is rich in vitamins, calcium, potassium and other minerals matter. It can be fried and cooked with necessary ingredients. The tender fruit can be cut into small pieces, boiled and served with soup. Matured fruit and stems containing crude fibre are used in the paper industry.

Okra (Abelmoschus esculentus L) is commonly known as bhindi or lady's finger belonging to family Malvaceae. It is an important fruit vegetable crop cultivated in various states of India. Several species of the genus Abelmoschus are grown in many parts of the world among them Abelmoschus esculentus is most commonly cultivated in Asia and has a great commercial demand due to its nutritional values.

The genus Abelmoschus was established by Medikus in 1787. However most authors followed deCandolle (1883) and treated it as a section of Hibiscus. It was Hochreutiner in 1924, who reinstated the genus Abelmoschus of Medikus, stating that calyx, corolla and stamens are fused together at the base and fall as one piece after anthesis whereas incase of Hibiscus these are distinct. Though the genus is of Asiatic origin, the origin of cultigen A.

esculentus has been reported to be variable from India; Ethiopia, West Africa and Tropical Asia. However, Zeven and Zhukovasky, 1975 believed it to have originated from India. This view is strengthened from the Sanskrit words, Tindisha and Gandhmula found to designate Bhindi. Thus it is likely that the cultigen might have originated in Asia or it might originally have been present in Africa and India as a polyphyletic species. Again there is not much evidence available to show as to when and how cultivated Bhindi got introduced in India. There is no mention in 'Ain-e-Akbari' or any other archeological records. This shows that it does not have a long history of cultivation in this country. Probably it reached India by the end of 19th century.

# PREGNANCY

The state of carrying a developing embryo or fetus within the female body. This condition can be indicated by positive results on an over-the-counter urine test, and confirmed through a blood test, ultrasound, detection of fetal heartbeat, or an X-ray. Pregnancy lasts for about nine months, measured from the date of the woman's last menstrual period (LMP). It is conventionally divided into three trimesters, each roughly three months long.

The most important tasks of basic fetal cell differentiation occur during the first trimester, so any harm done to the fetus during this period is most likely to result in miscarriage or serious disability. There is little to no chance that a first-trimester fetus can survive outside the womb, even with the best hospital care. Its systems are simply too undeveloped. This stage truly ends with the phenomenon of quickening: the mother's first perception of fetal movement. It is in the first trimester that some women experience "morning sickness," a form of nausea on awaking that usually passes within an hour. The breasts also begin to prepare for nursing, and painful soreness from hardening milk glands may result. As the pregnancy progresses, the mother may experience many physical and emotional changes, ranging from increased moodiness to darkening of the skin in various areas. During the second trimester, the fetus undergoes a remarkable series of developments. Its physical parts become fully distinct and at least somewhat operational. With the best medical care, a second-trimester fetus born prematurely has at least some chance of survival, although developmental delays and other handicaps may emerge later. As the fetus grows in size, the mother's pregnant state will begin to be obvious. In the third trimester, the fetus enters the final stage of preparation for birth. It increases rapidly in weight, as does the mother. As the end of the pregnancy nears, there may be discomfort as the fetus moves into position in the woman's lower abdomen. Edema (swelling of the ankles), back pain, and balance problems are sometimes experienced during this time period. Most women are able to go about their usual activities until the very last days or weeks of pregnancy, including non-impact exercise and work. During the final days, some feel too much discomfort to continue at a full pace, although others report greatly increased energy just before the birth. Pregnancy ends when the birth process begins.

See also acute fatty liver of pregnancy; ectopic pregnancy; fetal alcohol syndrome; fetal alcohol effect; hyperemesis gravidarum; preeclampsia; pregnancy, tubal; prenatal care; prenatal development; birth defect; teratogen.

# The Three Stages of Pregnancy (1st, 2nd, and 3rd Trimester)

Conception to about the 12th week of pregnancy marks the first trimester. The second trimester is weeks 13 to 27, and the third trimester starts about 28 weeks and lasts until birth. This slide show will discuss what occurs to both the mother and baby during each trimester.

First Trimester

First Trimester: Week 1 (conception) – Week 12

First Trimester: Early Changes in a Woman's Body

The early changes that signify pregnancy become present in the first trimester. A missed period may be the first sign that fertilization and implantation have occurred, ovulation has ceased, and you are pregnant. Other changes will also occur.

First Trimester: Physical and Emotional Changes a Woman May Experience

Hormonal changes will affect almost every organ in the body. Some signs of early pregnancy in many women include symptoms like:

- Extreme fatigue
- Tender, swollen breasts. Nipples may protrude.
- Nausea with or without throwing up (morning sickness)
- Cravings or aversion to certain foods
- Mood swings
- Constipation
- Frequent urination
- Headache
- Heartburn
- Weight gain or loss

First Trimester: Changes in a Woman's Daily Routine

Some of the changes you experience in your first trimester may cause you to revise your daily routine. You may need to go to bed earlier or eat more frequent or smaller meals. Some women experience a lot of discomfort, and others may not feel any at all. Pregnant women experience pregnancy differently and even if they've been pregnant before. Pregnant women may feel completely differently with each subsequent pregnancy.

First Trimester: The Baby at 4 Weeks

At 4 weeks, your baby is developing:

- The nervous system (brain and spinal cord) has begun to form.
- The heart begins to form.
- Arm and leg buds begin to develop.
- Your baby is now an embryo and 1/25 of an inch long.

First Trimester: The Baby at 8 Weeks

At 8 weeks, the embryo begins to develop into a fetus. Fetal development is apparent:

- All major organs have begun to form.
- The baby's heart begins to beat.
- The arms and legs grow longer.
- Fingers and toes have begun to form.
- Sex organs begin to form.
- The face begins to develop features.
- The umbilical cord is clearly visible.
- At the end of 8 weeks, your baby is a fetus, and is nearly 1 inch long, weighing less than ⅛ of an ounce.

First Trimester: The Baby at 12 Weeks

The end of the first trimester is at about week 12, at this point in your baby's development:

- The nerves and muscles begin to work together. Your baby can make a fist.
- The external sex organs show if your baby is a boy or girl.
- Eyelids close to protect the developing eyes. They will not open again until week 28.
- Head growth has slowed, and your baby is about 3 inches long, and weighs almost an ounce.

**Second Trimester**

Second trimester: Week 13 – Week 28

Second Trimester: Changes a Woman May Experience

Once you enter the second trimester you may find it easier than the first. Your nausea (morning sickness) and fatigue may lessen or go away completely. However, you will also notice more changes to your body. That "baby bump" will start to show as your abdomen expands with the growing baby. By the end of the second trimester you will even be able to feel your baby move!

Second Trimester: Physical and Emotional Changes in a Woman

Some changes you may notice in your body in the second trimester include:

- Back, abdomen, groin, or thigh aches and pains
- Stretch marks on your abdomen, breasts, thighs, or buttocks
- Darkening of the skin around your nipples
- A line on the skin running from belly button to pubic hairline (linea nigra)
- Patches of darker skin, usually over the cheeks, forehead, nose, or upper lip. This is sometimes called the mask of pregnancy (melasma, or Chloasma facies).
- Numb or tingling hands (carpal tunnel syndrome)
- Itching on the abdomen, palms, and soles of the feet. (Call your doctor if you have nausea, loss of appetite, vomiting, yellowing of skin, or fatigue combined with itching. These can be signs of a liver problem.)
- Swelling of the ankles, fingers, and face. (If you notice any sudden or extreme swelling or if you gain a lot of weight quickly, call your doctor immediately. This could be a sign of a serious condition called preeclampsia.)

Second Trimester: The Baby at 16 Weeks

As your body changes in the second trimester, your baby continues to develop:

- The musculoskeletal system continues to form.
- Skin begins to form and is nearly translucent.
- Meconium develops in your baby's intestinal tract. This will be your baby's first bowel movement.
- Your baby begins sucking motions with the mouth (sucking reflex).
- Your baby is about 4 to 5 inches long and weighs almost 3 ounces.

Second Trimester: The Baby at 20 Weeks

At about 20 weeks in the second trimester, your baby continues to develop:

- Your baby is more active. You might feel movement or kicking.
- Your baby is covered by fine, feathery hair called lanugo and a waxy protective coating called vernix.
- Eyebrows, eyelashes, fingernails, and toenails have formed. Your baby can even scratch itself.
- Your baby can hear and swallow.
- Now halfway through your pregnancy, your baby is about 6 inches long and weighs about 9 ounces.

Second Trimester: The Baby at 24 Weeks

By 24 weeks, even more changes occur for your growing baby:

- The baby's bone marrow begins to make blood cells.
- Taste buds form on your baby's tongue.
- Footprints and fingerprints have formed.
- Hair begins to grow on your baby's head.
- The lungs are formed, but do not yet work.
- Your baby has a regular sleep cycle.
- If your baby is a boy, his testicles begin to descend into the scrotum. If your baby is a girl, her uterus and ovaries are in place, and a lifetime supply of eggs has formed in the ovaries.
- Your baby stores fat and weighs about 1½ pounds, and is 12 inches long.

## Third Trimester

Third Trimester: Week 29 – Week 40 (birth)

Third Trimester: Changes a Woman May Experience

The third trimester is the final stage of pregnancy. Discomforts that started in the second trimester will likely continue, along with some new ones. As the baby grows and puts more pressure on your internal organs, you may find you have difficulty breathing and have to urinate more frequently. This is normal and once you give birth these problems should go away.

Third Trimester: Emotional and Physical Changes a Woman May Experience

In the third and final trimester you will notice more physical changes, including:

- Swelling of the ankles, fingers, and face. (If you notice any sudden or extreme swelling or if you gain a lot of weight really quickly, call your doctor right away. This could be a sign of a serious condition called preeclampsia.)
- Hemorrhoids
- Tender breasts, which may leak a watery pre-milk called colostrum
- Your belly button may protrude
- The baby "dropping," or moving lower in your abdomen
- Contractions, which can be a sign of real or false labor
- Other symptoms you may notice in the third trimester include shortness of breath, heartburn, and difficulty sleeping

Third Trimester: Changes as the Due Date Approaches

Other changes are happening in your body during the third trimester that you can't see. As your due date approaches, your cervix becomes thinner and softer in a process called effacement that helps the cervix open during childbirth. Your doctor will monitor the progress of your pregnancy with regular exams, especially as you near your due date.

Third Trimester: The Baby at 32 Weeks

At 32 weeks in the third trimester, your baby's development continues:

- Your baby's bones are soft but fully formed.
- Movements and kicking increase.
- The eyes can open and close.
- Lungs are not fully formed, but practice "breathing" movements occur.
- Your baby's body begins to store vital minerals, such as iron and calcium.
- Lanugo (fine hair) begins to fall off.
- Your baby is gaining about ½ pound a week, weighs about 4 to 4½ pounds, and is about 15 to 17 inches long.

Third Trimester: The Baby at 36 Weeks

At 36 weeks, as your due date approaches, your baby continues development:

- The protective waxy coating (vernix) thickens.
- Body fat increases.
- Your baby is getting bigger and has less space to move around. Movements are less forceful, but you will still feel them.
- Your baby is about 16 to 19 inches long and weighs about 6 to 6½ pounds.

Third Trimester: The baby at 37 to 40 Weeks

Finally, from 37 to 40 weeks the last stages of your baby's development occur:

- By the end of 37 weeks, your baby is considered full term.
- Your baby's organs are capable of functioning on their own.
- As you near your due date, your baby may turn into a head-down position for birth.

- Average birth weight is between 6 pounds 2 ounces to 9 pounds 2 ounces and average length is 19 to 21 inches long. Most full-term babies fall within these ranges, but healthy babies come in many different weights and sizes.

## Symptoms of Pregnancy

Every woman is different. So are her experiences of pregnancy. Not every woman has the same symptoms or even the same symptoms from one pregnancy to the next.

Also, because the early symptoms of pregnancy often mimic the symptoms you might experience right before and during menstruation, you may not realize you're pregnant.

What follows is a description of some of the most common early symptoms of pregnancy. You should know that these symptoms may be caused by other things besides being pregnant. So the fact that you notice some of these symptoms does not necessarily mean you are pregnant. The only way to tell for sure is with a pregnancy test.

**Spotting and Cramping**

After conception, the fertilized egg attaches itself to wall of the uterus. This can cause one of the earliest signs of pregnancy -- spotting and, sometimes, cramping.

That's called implantation bleeding. It occurs anywhere from six to 12 days after the egg is fertilized.

The cramps resemble menstrual cramps, so some women mistake them and the bleeding for the start of their period. The bleeding and cramps, however, are slight.

Besides bleeding, a woman may notice a white, milky discharge from her vagina. That's related to the thickening of the vagina's walls, which starts almost immediately after conception. The increased growth of cells lining the vagina causes the discharge.

This discharge, which can continue throughout pregnancy, is typically harmless and doesn't require treatment. But if there is a bad smell related to the discharge or a burning and itching sensation, tell your doctor so they can check on whether you have a yeast or bacterial infection.

## Breast Changes

Breast changes are another very early sign of pregnancy. A woman's hormone levels rapidly change after conception. Because of the changes, her breasts may become swollen, sore, or tingly a week or two later. Or they may feel heavier or fuller or feel tender to the touch. The area around the nipples, called the areola, may also darken.

Other things could cause breast changes. But if the changes are an early symptom of pregnancy, keep in mind that it is going to take several weeks to get used to the new levels of hormones. But when it does, breast pain should ease up.

## Fatigue

Feeling very tired is normal in pregnancy, starting early on.

A woman can start feeling unusually fatigued as soon as one week after conceiving.

Why? It's often related to a high level of a hormone called progesterone, although other things -- such as lower levels of blood sugar, lower blood pressure, and a boost in blood production -- can all contribute.

If fatigue is related to pregnancy, it's important to get plenty of rest. Eating foods that are rich in protein and iron can help offset it.

## Nausea (Morning Sickness)

Morning sickness is a famous symptom of pregnancy. But not every pregnant woman gets it.

The exact cause of morning sickness is not known but pregnancy hormones likely contribute to this symptom. Nausea during pregnancy may occur at any time of the day but most commonly in the morning.

Also, some women crave, or can't stand, certain foods when they become pregnant. That's also related to hormonal changes. The effect can be so strong that even the thought of what used to be a favorite food can turn a pregnant woman's stomach.

It's possible that the nausea, cravings, and food aversions can last for the entire pregnancy. Fortunately, the symptoms lessen for many women at about the 13th or 14th week of their pregnancy.

In the meantime, be sure to eat a healthy diet so that you and your developing baby get essential nutrients. You can talk to your doctor for advice on that.

## Missed Period

The most obvious early symptom of pregnancy -- and the one that prompts most women to get a pregnancy test -- is a missed period. But not all missed or delayed periods are caused by pregnancy.

Also, women can experience some bleeding during pregnancy. If you are pregnant, ask your doctor what you should be aware of with bleeding. For example, when is bleeding normal and when is it a sign of an emergency?

There are reasons, besides pregnancy, for missing a period. it might be that you gained or lost too much weight. Hormonal problems, fatigue, or stress are other possibilities. Some women miss their period when they stop taking birth control pills. But if a period is late and pregnancy is a possibility, you may want to get a pregnancy test.

## Causes of pregnancy

In order for pregnancy to happen, sperm needs to meet up with an egg. Pregnancy officially starts when a fertilized egg implants in the lining of the uterus. It takes up to 2-3 weeks after sex for pregnancy to happen.

Pregnancy is actually a pretty complicated process that has several steps. It all starts with sperm cells and an egg.

Sperm are microscopic cells that are made in testicles. Sperm mixes with other fluids to make semen (cum), which comes out of the penis during ejaculation. Millions and millions of sperm come out every time you ejaculate — but it only takes 1 sperm cell to meet with an egg for pregnancy to happen.

Eggs live in ovaries, and the hormones that control your menstrual cycle cause a few eggs to mature every month. When your egg is mature, it means it's ready to be fertilized by a sperm cell. These hormones also make the lining of your uterus thick and spongy, which gets your body ready for pregnancy.

About halfway through your menstrual cycle, one mature egg leaves the ovary — called ovulation — and travels through the fallopian tube towards your uterus.

The egg hangs out for about 12-24 hours, slowly moving through the fallopian tube, to see if any sperm are around.

If semen gets in the vagina, the sperm cells can swim up through the cervix and uterus and into the fallopian tubes, looking for an egg. They have up to 6 days to find an egg before they die.

When a sperm cell joins with an egg, it's called fertilization. Fertilization doesn't happen right away. Since sperm can hang out in your uterus and fallopian tube for up to 6 days after sex, there's up to 6 days between sex and fertilization.

If a sperm cell does join up with your egg, the fertilized egg moves down the fallopian tube toward the uterus. It begins to divide into more and more cells, forming a ball as it grows. The ball of cells (called a blastocyst) gets to the uterus about 3–4 days after fertilization.

The ball of cells floats in the uterus for another 2–3 days. If the ball of cells attaches to the lining of your uterus, it's called implantation — when pregnancy officially begins.

Implantation usually starts about 6 days after fertilization, and takes about 3-4 days to complete. The embryo develops from cells on the inside of the ball. The placenta develops from the cells on the outside of the ball.

When a fertilized egg implants in the uterus, it releases pregnancy hormones that prevent the lining of your uterus from shedding — that's why people don't get periods when they're pregnant. If your egg doesn't meet up with sperm, or a fertilized egg doesn't implant in your uterus, the thick lining of your uterus isn't needed and it leaves your body during your period. Up to half of all fertilized eggs naturally don't implant in the uterus — they pass out of your body during your period.

# Diagnosis

The diagnosis of pregnancy traditionally has been made from history and physical examination. Important aspects of the menstrual history must be obtained. The woman should describe her usual menstrual pattern, including date of onset of last menses, duration, flow, and frequency. Items that may confuse the diagnosis of early pregnancy are an atypical last menstrual period (LMP), contraceptive use, and history of irregular menses. Additionally, as many as 25% of women bleed during their first trimester, further complicating the assessment.

Be alert to the presentation of rising human chorionic gonadotropin (hCG) levels, an empty uterus observed on US, abdominal pain, and vaginal bleeding, as these may signal an ectopic pregnancy. Ectopic pregnancies are the number one cause of first trimester maternal mortality and should be diagnosed early, before the pregnancy ruptures or the patient becomes unstable . Other historical factors related to ectopic pregnancies include prior tubal manipulation, pelvic inflammatory disease (PID), previous ectopic pregnancy, tubal disease, use of an intrauterine device (IUD) for contraception, fertility therapies, and tubal ligation.

The classic presentation of pregnancy is a woman with menses of regular frequency who presents with amenorrhea, nausea, vomiting, generalized malaise, and breast tenderness.

Upon physical examination, one may find an enlarged uterus on bimanual exam, breast changes, and softening and enlargement of the cervix (Hegar sign; observed at approximately 6 wk). The Chadwick sign is a bluish discoloration of the cervix from venous congestion and can be observed by 8-10 weeks. A gravid uterus may be palpable low in the abdomen if the pregnancy has progressed far enough, usually by 12 weeks. Currently, through the use of chemical assays and US, physicians are capable of making the diagnosis of pregnancy before many of the physical signs and symptoms are evident.

With the advent of transvaginal ultrasound (TVUS), the diagnosis of pregnancy can be made even earlier than is capable with transabdominal scans. US has long been used in uncomplicated pregnancies for dating and as a screening exam for fetal anomalies. US typically is not used to diagnose pregnancy unless the patient presents with vaginal bleeding or abdominal pain early in gestation or is a high-risk obstetric patient. TVUS is the most accurate means of confirming intrauterine pregnancy and gestational age during the early first trimester.

TVUS has several advantages over transabdominal ultrasound (TAUS) during early pregnancy. TVUS can detect signs of intrauterine pregnancy approximately 1 week earlier than TAUS. Patients are not required to have a full bladder and are not required to endure uncomfortable pressure on the abdominal wall from the external probe. TVUS also is better when approaching patients who are obese or those who guard during TAUS examination. On the down side, some patients are anxious about the transvaginal probe and may object to its insertion.

Vaginal probes typically are higher frequency (5-8 MHz) than abdominal probes (3-5 MHz). The higher frequency allows for better resolution of the image but less penetration. Also, practice is necessary for familiarization with the orientation on the US monitor when performing TVUS.

The earliest structure identified is the gestational sac (GS). The GS can be seen on TVUS by 4-5 weeks' gestation and grows at a rate of 1 mm/d in early gestation. By 5.5-6 weeks, a double-decidual sign can be seen, which is the GS surrounded by the thickened decidua. The presence of an early GS can be confused with a small collection of fluid or blood or the pseudogestational sac of an ectopic pregnancy. Because of this, the diagnosis of intrauterine pregnancy should not be made with visualization of the GS alone.

The yolk sac can be recognized by 4-5 weeks' gestation and is seen until approximately 10 weeks?gestation. The yolk sac is a small sphere with a hypoechoic center and is located within the GS . Observing a GS that is larger 10 mm without a yolk sac is rare, and if this is observed, it most likely represents an abnormal pregnancy . Likewise, a yolk sac larger than 7 mm without evidence of a developing fetal pole suggests a nonviable pregnancy. The diagnosis of intrauterine pregnancy can be made once the yolk sac is present, which also rules out an ectopic pregnancy, except in the rare instance of heterotopic pregnancy. Heterotopic pregnancy, an intrauterine pregnancy, and an ectopic pregnancy during the same gestation was once thought to be extremely rare but now has been shown to be present in as many as 1 per 3000 pregnancies.

The fetal or embryonic pole is first seen on TVUS at approximately 5-6 weeks?gestation. The fetal pole is a linear hyperechoic structure that grows at approximately 1 mm/d. Cardiac motion sometimes can be identified in a 2- to 3-mm embryo but almost always is present when the embryo grows to 5 mm or longer.

## OKRA

Okra is a warm-season vegetable, also known as gumbo or ladies' fingers. It is a good source of minerals, vitamins, and fiber. It contains a characteristic viscous juice that can be used to thicken sauces.

Gumbo is popular in the southern United States (U.S.), parts of Africa and the Middle East, the Caribbean, and South America.

It is considered an important crop in many countries, because of its nutritional value, and because many parts of the plant can be used, including the fresh leaves, buds, flowers, pods, stems, and seeds.

The taste is mild, but it has a unique texture with peach-like fuzz on the outside and small, edible seeds on the inside of the pod.

It offers a wide range of health benefits.

We will look at the nutritional content of okra, its possible health benefits, recipe tips for preparing okra, and any possible health risks.

## The Benefits Of Okra During Pregnancy

The nutrients present in okra are very beneficial for pregnancy and aid in the healthy development of the baby. Read on to know more about the benefits that okra has to offer.

1. Contain vitamin C: Vitamin C helps in the absorption of iron, which promotes the growth of the baby. It also boosts immunity of the mother and promotes the development of skin, bones, and capillaries in the baby (2).

2. High in folate: Okra is a potent source of folate, which lowers the risk of birth defects in the baby. It also boosts the metabolism of carbs, protein and fat, and helps synthesize DNA and red blood cells (3).

3. A source of antioxidants: The major antioxidants in okra include carotenoids, phenolic compounds, vitamins C and E. They promote the mother's and baby's immune system, and therefore lower the chances of any infections and cardiovascular issues (1).

4. Contain fiber: Rich in both soluble and insoluble fiber, okra helps in abating constipation during pregnancy. Soluble fiber works to lower blood cholesterol and treats diabetes, and insoluble fiber promotes digestion (4).

5. Okra is not known to cause any side effects during pregnancy, which makes it a vegetable that you must include in your diet during pregnancy.
6. Keep reading for a breakdown of the nutrients in this vegetable.

## Nutritional Value Of Okra

Nutrients present in 100 grams of okra are as follows (5):

| NUTRIENT | AMOUNT |
|---|---|
| Calories | 33kcal |
| Water | 89.58g |
| Carbohydrates | 7.45g |
| Sugars | 1.48g |
| Protein | 1.93g |
| Fiber | 3.2g |
| Fat | 0.19g |
| Vitamins | |
| Thiamin (Vitamin B1) | 0.200mg |
| Riboflavin (Vitamin B2) | 0.060mg |
| Niacin (Vitamin B3) | 1mg |
| Pyridoxine (Vitamin B6) | 0.215mg |
| Folic acid (Vitamin B9) | 60mcg |
| Ascorbic acid (Vitamin C) | 23mg |
| Retinol (Vitamin A) | 716U |
| Alpha-tocopherol (Vitamin E) | 0.27mg |

| | |
|---|---|
| Phylloquinone (Vitamin K) | 31.3mcg |
| Electrolytes | |
| Potassium | 299mg |
| Sodium | 7mg |
| Minerals | |
| Calcium | 82mg |
| Iron | 0.62mg |
| Phosphorus | 61mg |
| Magnesium | 57mg |
| Zinc | 0.58mg |
| Lipids | |
| Total saturated fatty acids | 0.026g |
| Total monounsaturated fatty acids | 0.017g |
| Total polyunsaturated fatty acids | 0.027g |

In the following section, we tell you how to include okra in your pregnancy diet, along with a few easy recipes that you can try.

## OKRA FOR PREGNANT WOMAN

Okra, also known as ladies' finger or ochro, is grown in tropical and warm temperate parts of the world. The vegetable is available throughout the year, but the best produce is available during the early spring season. Its nutritional goodness has made it a part of pregnancy diet in various regions of the world. Here, MomJunction tells you about the benefits of eating okra during pregnancy, its nutritional value, and ways to include it in your diet.

okra is a nutritious pod vegetable that is good to eat during pregnancy. It is rich in fiber, folic acid, protein, carbohydrate, Vitamin C, B3, and K, beta-carotene, potassium, calcium, and phosphorus. Whether you eat it boiled, stewed, fried or pickled, you will be able to benefit from the nutrients it has (1).

Ways to Include Okra in Pregnancy Diet

Here are some tips and precautions for including okra in your diet.

- Rinse okra thoroughly before cooking it. It minimizes any risk of infection.

- Cook on low flame to prevent loss of nutrients.

- Make delicious finger food by slitting the vegetable in half, coating with gram flour and frying in oil.

- Frying sliced okra, coated with breadcrumbs, is another way to consume okra.

- Crush two okras and soak in a glass of water overnight. Consume the water next morning for detoxification and regulating cholesterol levels.

## Dosage

- Keep okra dry, and do not wash it until you are ready to use it. Storing it in the crisper drawer in a paper or plastic bag can stop it becoming slimy or moldy. Fresh okra does not last for more than 3 to 4 days.

- Ladies' fingers can be used in salads, soups, and stews, fresh or dried, fried, sautéed, roasted, or boiled. They can also be pickled.
- Cutting okra and cooking it in moisture releases a mucilaginous, or slimy, juice that increases the thickness of soups and stews. Dried okra can also be used to make or thicken a sauce, or as an egg white substitute.
- Okra seeds can also be roasted and ground to make a non-caffeinated coffee substitute.
- Some people do not enjoy the gummy texture of okra. Cooking the whole pods quickly can avoid this.

# Side Effects

Eating too much okra can have an adverse effect on some people.

Fructans and gastrointestinal problems: Okra is rich in fructans, a type of carbohydrate that can cause diarrhea, gas, cramping, and bloating in people with bowel problems. People with irritable bowel syndrome (IBS) and other gut conditions are more likely to be sensitive to foods high in fructans.

Oxalates and kidney stones: Okra is also high in oxalates. The most common type of kidney stone is made of calcium oxalate.

According to the National Institute of Diabetes and Digestive and Kidney Diseases (NDDKD), high-oxalate foods can increase the risk of these stones in people who have had them previously. Other high oxalate foods include spinach, rhubarb, and Swiss chard.

Solanine and inflammation: Okra contains a compound called solanine. Solanine is a toxic chemical that has been linked to joint pain, arthritis, and long-lasting inflammation for a small percentage of people who may be sensitive to it. It is found in many fruits and vegetables, including potatoes, tomatoes, eggplant, blueberries, and artichokes.

No studies have suggested reducing solanine intake for the general population. In general, vegetables and fruits help reduce inflammation.

Vitamin K and blood clotting: Okra, and other foods that are high in vitamin K, can affect those who use blood-thinning drugs like warfarin, or Coumadin. Blood thinners are used to prevent harmful blood clots that can block blood from getting to the brain or heart.

Vitamin K helps the blood to clot. People who are at risk of blood clots should not suddenly change the amount of vitamin K they eat but keep their intake of vitamin-K-rich foods steady from day to day.

Made in the USA
Monee, IL
09 April 2022